Bursting with Danger
and Music

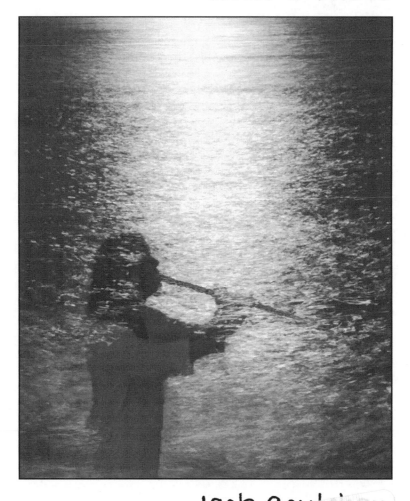

Jack Coulehan

Plain View Press
http://plainviewpress.net

...00 N. Lamar, Suite 730-260
Austin, TX 78756

ISBN: 978-1-935514-84-8
Library of Congress Control Number: 2011945368

Cover art: Virginia Bushart
Cover design by Pam Knight

To my grandchildren,

Jack

Cate

Collin

and

Addison

Acknowledgements

I am grateful for permission to reprint the following poems, many of which appeared in earlier forms and/or with different titles:

Journal of the American Medical Association (JAMA)—"The Act of Love," "Babushka," "Balancing Books," "Cosmic Sonnets," "Darkness Is Gathering Me," "Deep Structures," "Do No Harm," "Ghazal on Miracles," "Grackles," "In Praise of Virtue," "Levitation," "Lillian's Vision," "Lovesickness," "Nesidioblastosis," "Phrenology," "Pit Bill," "Predators," "Sweetness," "Sewage Treatment," "Snoring," "Soundings: Three for the Stethoscope," "Swimming," "Tattoos," "A Theory of Labor," "Ultrasound," "Why I Am Not a Pathologist," and "The Words."

Annals of Internal Medicine—"Astonishment," "Cockroach," "Detached Concern," "Empty Soup," "He Lectures on Grace," "Geode," "The Goddess Grabs Me by the Hair," "Interned," "Joys and Delights, Griefs and Despondencies," "A Mission of Mercy," "Midnight Supper," and "That Intern Dream."

The Pharos—"Virginia Ham" and "Forbidden Perfume."

Canadian Medical Association Journal—"The Poor Historian" and "William Carlos Williams Circumcises Hemingway's First Son."

The Lancet, "Isn't"

Other credits— "Theology" in *Bellevue Literary Review*; "The Letter" in *Birmingham Poetry Review*; "Funny, All I Can Think About Is Sin" in *California Quarterly*; "To the Man With the Video Camera at the Monastery on Patmos" in *Comstock Review*; "Five Moons of Venus" in *Connecticut River Review*; "The The Invention of Language" in *Freshwater*; "Slipping Away" in *The Healing Muse*; "Absolution" in *International Journal of Healthcare*; "Banana Bread" and "Bursting With Danger and Music" in *Kansas Quarterly*; "Phantom Limb" in *Nimrod*; "Levitation" in *Poetry East*; "Heart Blockages" in *Potato Eyes*; "Phrenology" in *Rattle*; "Delicate Procedures" in *Oyez Review*; "The Little Flower" in *Rhode Island Writers Annual*; "All Souls' Day" in *South Coast Poetry Review*; "Darwin's Barnacles" in *Ulitarra (Australia)*; and "VACANCY" in *Widener Review*.

Earlier versions of several of these poems previously appeared in *The Knitted Glove*, *First Photographs of Heaven*, or *The Heavenly Ladder*.

Contents

Deep Structures   9

All Souls' Day   29

After Chekhov 49

He Lectures on Grace 63

Levitation 77

Natural History 93

Deep Structures

Virginia Ham ✳

December isn't the same
since Mary Johnson's ham
packed in Styrofoam and ice

with packets of pancake mix
and slabs of frozen bacon
has stopped arriving.

A furnace in Mary's chest
had burned so fiercely hot, I swore
she wouldn't last that year,

let alone the next. And next.
By chance or prayer, but not
by me, the passion

of her white cells lessened,
the fire staunched, and she
began to breathe again.

It wasn't long till Mary ran
from our slagheap town
to a condo on the coast.

For thirteen years the ham,
steaming with dioxide ice,
appeared on my porch

around December first,
until instead its absence came
and said she'd gone.

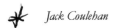

Jack Coulehan

The Act of Love

How foolish Celia must look
to the Haitian cab driver
on the Medicaid run!

She wears a white communion dress
the week before Easter, a sign
she brings me something more pressing

than the pain in her shoulder
and the son who doesn't talk to her
because his wife is embarrassed.

Her hips creak in conversation,
her knees grind, but even crepitant joints
are modestly silent and stand aside

when Celia hands me a potted plant
for my office—*an act of Christian love,*
she says, *not a sign of being personal.*

As for me, I'm stunned
out of the ordinary anger
at failing to help her

by the waxy-leaves of her gesture
and I receive this wafer of the season,
heartbroken for no reason.

Pit Bull

In a clinic constructed
of ugliness, I listen
to the pauses between
your outbursts about
the bad rap you didn't
deserve but God gave,
which proves he doesn't
exist or care, and the
insulin you don't take
because it makes you sick.

In your pierced face
with its ferocious
ornaments, I see
a ghostly embankment
near the Stony Brook
trestle, six months or more
after two girls from your class
guzzled wine with Xanax
in the weeds and dived
into the headlights
of an approaching train,

a story I've forgotten
until you come to the clinic—
hopeless, brittle, depressed,
your grief chained
and snarling. Cur,
bastard dog, get out
of her! Get out of that girl!

Jack Coulehan

Geode

I've come in time to miss seeing you
this morning. A crisp sheet, empty.
Your pillow puffed without depression.
With a bit of luck when you get back
from radiation, you'll fall so soundly
asleep, I'll miss you again this afternoon.

Just look at the clutter on your table:
that black comb you drag compulsively
through what's left of your hair, a box of taffy
from your office, a book about Major
John Wesley Powell and a Mexican geode,
sliced in half. Your niece's tinny voice

confessed to me she's finished. *What a loser
the man is!* You tossed her from the room
and now she won't come back until hell
freezes over. *Jealous, that's what he is,
the old fart.* Your geode, intractably dull
on the surface, captures my fingers.

What am I doing, poking around in this?
I can't remember the last time I stopped
and held a rock to the light, no reason—
the luminous quartz garden transforms
the rest of it—your chipped comb, the book,
my brilliant morning. I'm glad you're gone.

The Words

For the third time this month
his bronzed face
sits with its swaggering list

of what he needs me for—the test
he read about in Sunday's Times,
a second script for Vicodin

in case the pain that's almost gone
comes back, why his appetite
is shot, whether a drink at night

would do him good. That body
bears the years with regal grace.
That face is Olympian,

commanding and ageless—
the father of the gods
transformed into a futures

broker, a wheeler-dealer.
That immaculate sun-drenched chest
almost tugs me to his feet

to learn the secret of success
but I hold fast. That newest test
won't help either of us

nor will the trip to a clinic in Texas,
no matter how famous.
I want to escape from the room,

to leave him with his power
and run from mine, the words that cut
to his core: *Behold the pancreas!*

He looks at me with faint unease
rising in the creases of his eyes—
My words will make him mortal, he will die.

Jack Coulehan

Doctor's Absolution Poem

When they aren't sick, I schedule them back
in a few months to refurbish their pills
for pressure and sugar and water. I check
their labs and urines, but minimize frills…
in media res. Most of the visit
we talk about bosses, bosses' vengeance,
prancing office scum who make illicit
screwball passes, big shots, the innocents
who get shot down, their gardens, the old timers
who shoot-off about managing their wives
but manage to loose them, and the whiners,
the rumbas, the Jesus-is-my-Savior lives—
I sit behind my screen and listen.
Ego te absolvo doesn't hurt them.

Soundings: Three for the Stethoscope

1.

Let me place
these miniature pears
in my ears, this diaphragm
against your skin.

Listen—the wafting
of a cracked Victrola's voice
in the leaves of your garden.

2.

Wafting? What a word
for a simple
sonic phenomenon.

Leaves? I better stick
to the facts.
The noise is turbulence.

Garden? From plastic tubes
around my neck
a bell-shaped tuber.

3.

I slide the tuber
to the curve of your breast—

a waft of thuds and turbulence
instead of blips,
the scratch of tissue, this.

In an age of perfect machines,
how impertinent
to choose imperfect means!

Jack Coulehan

At Night the Sick Knock

I am the first guest
in a house so new its walls
bark at night.

In this fresh room,
the sap still rising in its boards,
I hear

the staccato knock of a drunk,
dead drunk, demanding medicine
at midnight,

a mother's tap in the dark,
her children sick, her babies wrapped.
Open up!

Let me in! Their voices crack.
Sound my baby.
Stitch his scalp.

In my own familiar house,
the nighttime knocks are distant,
deep, asleep.

But in this thin house,
the knocks
are knuckles at my ear—

the naked doors are hollow,
crack like tinder,
snap like beans.

I hear that midnight drunk
inside me,
Let me in!

Douse my fever.
Soothe my skin.

Ghazal on Miracles

Nothing less than a miracle will do. Nothing less
than dowsing disbelief. Nothing more, nothing less.

Take the terrified woman who failed to respond
to chemo. She anticipated more and never less.

Is it wise to embrace morphine's unsteadiness,
itch, and confusion? Or is hoping better with less?

Take only yes for an answer. Never say never,
even in winter, or later. For nothing is less.

Cycles of chemo fire up the engines of success.
Is it miraculous? Could it never be less?

Miracle of compassion. Miracle of grace.
Miracle to suffer more for the sake of less.

Nothing happens that hasn't recurred. Nothing is given
without disguise, neither a miracle, nor anything less.

Jack Coulehan

Swimming

She'll always be diving
into the Schuylkill River,
surviving until I get there,

and showing the six months'
sweet rise of her womb,
and the fetus, for all I know,

will cry out for justice,
if not for love, when I arrive
in the ER to check her.

My brain will always be
on its own, drifting elsewhere
with moisture in its hair.

I suppose she'll always be
grabbing my arm and screaming
about the voices and terror

as I listen to her heart.
And none of the units
at Philadelphia General

will take her, so I'll send her
out to the State again,
assigned to a suicide watch.

The last I'll see is her gurney
pushed by the back of a cop
to the ambulance dock.

And, of course, her brain
will always begin to bleed
as she's swimming out.

Balancing Books

> *"If you want to die you will have to pay for it."*
> Louis MacNeice, "Charon"

You roll into the room flat on a bed
with a screen winking above your shoulder.

Light penetrates the sheets of a niche
where they put you, awaiting the tug

of hope and the deep drag of flesh
to play themselves out. Too much clutter

to reflect, too many branches to cut,
your loader pushes and drips, your drainer

relieves the pressure. The body
scribbles in diminishing letters,

speaks in whispers, misplaces your thread.
Which is the right place? You had meant

to ask at the gate, but before you could
they clapped a charge on your chest. They looked

at your heart's account and said, *If you want
to die, you will have to pay for it.*

Jack Coulehan

Deep Structures

I never knew how deep the structures were
or why the names for them intrigued me so.
Amygdaloid—the sound tripped off my tongue.
And *hippocampal gyrus* made me sing.

The music of these names intrigues me so,
though the tendons of my hand—forgotten all.
And *hippocampal gyrus* makes me sing,
for thirty years still dancing from my tongue.

The tendons of my hand—forgotten all,
as are the layered structures of my back.
Yet thirty years of tumbling off my tongue—
those rhythmic nebulae within my brain.

The muscled structures of my back are zip.
But *caudate, red,* and *pallidum* survive—
those rhythmic nebulae that strum my brain.
Gone, passion that I had for listing names.

But *caudate, red,* and *pallidus* endure,
and *amygdaloid*, an almost perfect self.
Gone, passion for obsessive naming names,
but those archaic structures still grip firm.

Amygdaloid is almost perfect self.
And even though I judged my soul was lost,
those deep archaic structures never budged,
but form the links by which our lives connect.

And even though I judged my soul was lost
I never knew how deep its structures were,
their buried links by which our lives connect.
Amygdaloid! It dances from my tongue.

The Internship Sonnets

1. Orientation

Orientation. He appeared at seven,
welcomed by a voice, *You don't belong,*
a repetitive warning that no one
heard but him. The Chief arose. A strong
odor of eagerness arrived. The other
interns smiled and shrugged, their faces eased
by conversation, a band of brothers
being forged. He looked down, took a piece
of paper and scribbled, *I'm terrified*
to start. How about you? But put it between
some pages. Whom to trust? Could he rely
on their eye contact? His neighbors' keen
gazes slid by. Not one of them saw him.
He chose to keep his feelings hidden.

2. The Golden Rule

The first rule of the service: pledging
allegiance to the chief. Violations,
like telling patients the truth, or hedging
on unneeded tests, or taking vacations
from the floor, were dealt with severely.
The chief said, *Honey, the surgeons got it all.*
A piece of cake. Said, *Stan, you nearly*
died, but everything's fine. It was small,
nothing to worry. The chief discreetly
withdrew. After which, his patients burst
into, *So I'm cured?* Their fear, neatly
brushed aside. To whom was the intern's first
duty? Continents of pain. Callow youth.
To the chief, to medicine, to truth?

Jack Coulehan

3. Midnight Supper

Cold spaghetti and thirty two ounces
of Coke at midnight supper. A littered
foursome, in which the quietest announced
he had another hit. The embittered
second stabbed his plastic tray with his pen.
The third intern shuffled through a stack
of index cards; his wife's father in Johnstown
had just died of cancer. The last attacked
a stale Portuguese roll with his fork.
Gears grinding, motors turning, but nothing
happening. The ozone-like smell of stale work.
Did they suffer from sleep deprivation?
Thirty-six on and twelve off, a sublime
method of learning the value of time.

4. The Poor Historian

The indigents were placed in open wards,
thirty-two beds, beneath a maze of rods
and drapes that slid across, unless ignored,
to create private space, or the façade
of privacy. First floor, men; women above.
Heads near the wall and feet adjacent
to the aisle. A umbrous gallery of
portraits hung above the beds. The complaisant
noblesse oblige of it all. During rounds,
the chief in charge, the doctors said *ma'am*
and *sir*, while scavenging beneath brown
skin for carrion. An objective exam,
nothing personal. *The patient is a poor
historian*, they groaned. This lacks a cure.

24

5. Interned

Interned: To be coerced into a camp
and made to work, because of who you are.
To be Japanese-American during the war
and considered a traitor. To be clamped
into preventive detention, as Boer
women and children were by British
soldiers. Incarcerated. Diminished.
An alien about to be sent. The score
was hospital, eleven months; interns,
zero. He thanked the Good Lord for gifts
of resilience, appetite, and the swift
embrace of sleep. After which, he returned
to the world with a jolt—knocked out of bed
by a buzzer. Inclement weather ahead.

6. The Prodigal Son

Seven-forty-five, the twenty-sixth of June,
and Elizabeth Bishop is on my desk.
At last the rumbling of the storm is gone.
Early twilight. Rest. Eight of the past
nine days it rained, almost a record,
but not quite. I'm feeling that surge
of grace a good day gives. In my restored
future, I can see genius emerge
and fortune soar beyond these rented rooms,
infested stairwell, and naked chandelier.
Elizabeth Bishop, in one of her poems,
has the prodigal son, at the end of his year
in a pig sty, returning. Look at me come.
After a long absence, I'm arriving home.

Jack Coulehan

That Intern Dream

I had that intern dream again last night,
white coat and pants, but decades older
than the group of docs I hadn't met.

In the middle of the scene, I kept
clutching a fear so tight, my smile was tin,
but I hadn't seen a single patient yet.

At midnight the rumpled interns ate
cold spaghetti, bread and juice. In a seat
across the room, I scanned their faces,

convinced they hadn't seen my grievous sin
of never having learned to put
a tube in place, or make an incision.

Instead I read my books. Emergency!
My name was called. A code. I had to run,
but didn't know in which direction.

The route I took was wrong, and I reversed.
My coat and shirt went down. My pants collapsed.
I skimmed along in underpants and socks.

The call was cardiac. If there had been
a chance of saving face, it went. The patient
gasped for breath, but I had never seen

a cath put in, or learned resuscitation.
Crowded around his bed stood eyes
that relished the confusion. Nothing

worked. And then the dream resolved
in gratitude: my own body, my own bed,
my secret still secure, nobody dead.

Joys and Delights, Griefs and Despondencies

"From nothing but the brain come joys and delights,
laughter and sports, griefs and despondencies."
Hippocrates, *On the Sacred Disease*

The inner voice that Socrates
said was god, but the Athenian state
decided was blasphemy,
could have been tracked, as it ran
across his brain, had he had a scan.

Ezekiel might have safely ignored
his vision of the heavenly throne,
avoided the burden of prophecy,
and prevented the scene from recurring,
had he had access to dopamine.

The spirit journey of a shaman.
The stigmatists' recurrent wounds.
Bernadette's virginal apparition.
Every manifestation a certain,
but subtle, neural lesion.

The evidence is overwhelming
that my illusion of an interior
being, whether he be sweet
or unsavory, in terror
or ecstasy, is electricity.

Tiny bags, filaments, conduits,
miniature selves, deep within you
lives my childhood friend. Should I
put my shoulder to the wheel of truth
and chase him out, or let him be?

All Souls' Day

Heart Blockages

Those white ragged lines
are what's left of my vessels,
damaged legs and old spurs
that jostle bareback
on that black bull of a heart,
my heart,
whose flanks on the overhead screen
are heaving and faltering.

I watch my arteries taper,
twist, crimp to a thread
in a blockage so tight
it's a wonder
the front of my heart hasn't died.

I remember the rodeo
in Wilcox, Arizona,

where, leaning on a jeep behind the bleachers,
I dipped snuff like a cowboy
and bragged I could ride all night
through the gap in those black mountains.

Jack Coulehan

Ultrasound

A charcoal spot on the fetal heart—
not so evident you'd notice it
at first, not with the perfect chalk-like sketch
of a body kicking and swimming
its way into life. But in the thoughtful pause
that follows the image, the doctor mentions—
as if she were sending you a note
about lunch, her hand draped on the doorknob—
a comment almost, but not entirely,
insignificant. A tube of blood,
a remark concerning the splitting
of chromosomes, a flash of brightness
in her voice—*It's not so bad; it's nothing,*
really. No point in your waiting and watching
and counting the signs that all is well,
so many of them, stacked against a single hint
of damage—for the image of chance
is stronger than reason, and more certain.

Forbidden Perfume

Antiseptics sweeten, but cannot disguise
the deep intensity of urine in a room
where Justin Daly lives. Accidents pile up
on every shift, bags leak, linens soil.
An aide dumps a stack of crusted clothes
in a canvas bin. A woman swabs the floor.
But Justin, a bald man strapped to his seat,
pays no attention. He savors the scent
of the newly macadamized road
to Southfield, Jamaica, and the graveyard
of the Seventh Day Adventist Church,
where his wife, or maybe his daughter, is buried.
Pimento. Hibiscus. Smell of savannah
dripping with rain; forbidden perfume.

Jack Coulehan

Banana Bread

Today, after all these months,
you're on the phone again
about the bread you promised
after Easter. You have the right
rotten bunch of bananas.
Your legs are down a little,
but not from the water pill.
Still too sick to get here
by yourself. You'd call a taxi
but the way a driver looked
at you last week ... at sixty
seven yet! Men have only
the one thing on their minds
and you're preserved. First time
you called you wouldn't pay
my bill—why should you?—all I do
is talk and give you pills.
Next time your legs were fat
as alabaster columns,
cold as granite. The next call
you wondered what I think
of women running wild, what
with birth control. The evil one
is in us all. The last call
you said I'd have that loaf
of warm banana bread
for Christmas. February.
April. This time there you are,
your legs warm as two
light loaves, risen and powdered.

Referral from Delores

Aside from the fleshy mole on her chin,
her face is featureless, which isn't true
but seems so, this late in the afternoon
with a storm about to break through.

She doesn't have a complaint, but rather
a note from Delores Hernandez,
an aide at the home, who says her odor
sickens the residents and causes us

to wonder if she suffers from gangrene
or something. Maybe it's intestinal gas
she leaks, it's so persistent. Anything
we try is futile. Mary was homeless

and we had to delouse her when she came
at Thanksgiving, but now she's continent
of urine, except at night. We gave her clean
undergarments this morning. We sent

her to a dermatologist, who said the scales
are just dry skin—all according to Delores.
Playing with a paperclip, Mary smells
like Jean Naté this afternoon, coolly fresh

in her shapeless smock. Maybe the home
has cause to complain, but today? Neither stain
nor effluvium. Mary lacks a voice
as well, but I don't think she's in pain

because she hums at me and pops her lips,
content as a skunk, another victim
of prejudice, whose pungent odor trips
when someone threatening moves in.

Jack Coulehan

Lillian's Vision

Wipe off your glass eye, Lillian,
with that hanky-rag of yours.
Wet smoke burns your natural eye
and streaks your face with tears.

Damp socks curl before your hearth,
wet pants sizzle on the chair.
You brace against your davenport
as cancer tugs you to the floor.

You testified and spoke in tongues
when Kathryn Kuhlman called your name.
Home from her revival tent,
you hear the frenzied tongues again.

And see them: flicking tongues of fire.
They touch your clothes, they smell like myrrh.
His tongue leaps up to touch your sore
in a frenzy of succor.

Before the cancer twists your spine
and grips your cartilage with pain,
you greet the Holy Lord whose tongue
plucks the tumor, makes you clean.

Pop-in your glass eye, Lillian.
Wake the children! Raise your voice!
In the gullet of this fire,
you'll find your passage and you'll pass.

All Souls' Day

So much depends on this frail old man
who lurches from his seat—*I'm next!*—
and works his cane across the room.

He purses his lips, like a clarinetist
leading a parade among the graves
on All Souls Day. So much depends

on the white elastic rim of shorts
that shows above his belt, on the cap
he swoops above his speckled scalp,

Hey, doc! I'm almost there! Whether
I pick up my instrument and dance
behind him, or spread my picnic

on a white sarcophagus, or just
carry my dead inside, so much
depends on this frail old man

who swivels his bad foot forward,
loudly chewing, almost swallowing
the sharp black notes of his clarinet.

Jack Coulehan

Darkness Is Gathering Me

On Lines by Alphonse Daudet

False spring is making its rounds this morning.
Darkness is gathering me into its lair.
It's twilight and my nurses are speaking—
You'd think they were talking about flowers.

Darkness is gathering me into its lair
but it isn't unpleasant. I imagine
it's morning, and my nurses are speaking
in a warm meadow. I have no business

imagining, but it's not unpleasant,
the way the nurses say, *It's a lovely wound…*
In that meadow, a wound has no business
turning a sulfurous color and dying.

The way the nurses talk, the lovely wound
is my morning, my body, my daffodils
abloom in sulfurous colors. I'm dying
but loveliness isn't. Let them run laughing

into the morning. My bloody daffodils
and sweetly rotting smell, what a case
of loveliness! I'll scamper, laugh
and hoot and dance in their wake.

Those sweetly-smelling nurses! My rotten case
is nailed shut. When the morphine wears off,
where will hooting and dancing be? At my wake?
Their bodies are firm; I wish I could touch them.

When the morphine wears off, they'll nail me shut.
False spring is making its rounds this morning.
Their bodies are firm; I wish I could touch them.
It's twilight and my nurses are speaking.

Slipping Away

I'm not saying I didn't die
when the blood to my brain
sputtered to nothing this morning,

but because it felt so good
with my pain gone, and the scene
in this hospital room

turned topsy-turvy, death
slipped in behind my back,
but then my sister came—I hadn't

heard her voice so tense in years—
and the doc explained
I'm dead despite my heartbeat.

She saw little sparks of the past
sputtering out of me,
which she began to build

into a convulsion of guilt—
what was the point of that?
For me the only difference

death made was release from being
pinned to my bed and a sudden
spurt of tolerance, but my sister

asked to sleep on my death
and decide about pulling the tube
in the morning. I'll be gone then—

I'm pouring through the pores
of this room, I'm already
feeling the jazz and hormones begin.

Jack Coulehan

Phantom Limb

I won it playing a game of cancer
on the ball of my thumb. The mole
was innocent until proven wrong.
The score teetered back and forth
like a devil's pact, until I won
my reward—an arm that isn't there,
the ghostly absence of symmetry.

The doctor says the arm is in my brain.
I feed it acetaminophen, codeine,
and Vicodin at four, eight and noon.
It needs them to maintain a sense
of self worth. Without pain, my limb
would be nothing. But because it burns,
it is. I'm like a man who won

a hundred thousand bucks a year
for twenty years. The next night he took
a dive from the roof. Saved from death
by chance, now he carries a load
of nothing. Nada. Zip. See what I mean?
I need to lean on a phantom arm
to shoulder my good fortune.

Tattoos

The telephone lineman whose tattoos
I so admired was less than thirty.
They encircled his arms from shoulder
to wrist, his chest from the base of his neck
to the muscular ridge of his belly—
serpents, women, even St. Francis
with his hands raised to bless the animals
he's preaching to. But nothing
on his copper-colored back—not one piece
of art emblazoned in a spot
the lineman couldn't see. Can you imagine
the weight of his Garden of Eden,
at the moment of transgression,
pressing against you? Men like him,
rejection or weakness never occurs to them
until it happens. He was completely
etched, except the stretch of his back
where on its surface was his future.

Jack Coulehan

Isn't

Let me see if I have this right
about what it isn't. It isn't
the sugar. It isn't the blood clot.
It isn't you're just not telling me
because you think I'm too far gone
and can't handle it. And mostly
it isn't what I think it is.

I say my kidney feels like a bad
punch, but you say, *No, it isn't*
the kidney. The kidney's the champ
of your body. I say my knees
buckle, my head reels, and you say,
Take one to keep calm and some
aspirin, but not on an empty
stomach. For God's sake, relax.

What you mean is—Get out!
I don't care about you. I don't
need you. But the monster
comes craning its popped eyes
at everyone sooner or later,
even you. So relax. I hope
when you feel its sour breath
at your back, I'll be there to say
there's nothing to fear, it isn't
the monster. And anyway, it's
too early to know. Come back
when it's bigger.

Detached Concern

My doctor's not engaged enough
to touch my hand. I wonder where
her feelings are, the human stuff.

My doctor doesn't take much guff
from wimps like me. Whatever care
she dredges up, it's not enough.

Detached concern is far from tough.
It's thin and weak and pulseless, bare.
And human feelings screw its stuff.

The pains I feel are fairly rough.
Detached, my doctor wouldn't dare
engage them. They're not clear enough

to measure with her scope and cuff.
Her brow is knit, her white coat there,
but touching? No. No human stuff.

This sickness wears me down. I slough
my hope, my sense of trust, aware
my doctor's not engaged enough.
She's blocked her feelings, done her stuff.

Jack Coulehan

Case History

Her story starts the month
her husband died, spirals backwards
to the year she spent in bed
when she was twelve and to the valve

that later turned to stone
and to the day, sometime the year
that Stan was born, a surgeon
slipped into her heart and cracked

the blockage, and her story
circulates again, and soon
her husband brings the turtle home
for Stan and flowers for his Sweets

who doesn't die, and Rhoda's five,
which reminds her of the month
her husband died and of the year
she spent out west with Stan,

until his place became too small
for unpacked crates and the clicking
of her teeth and far too warm
for all his talk about the women,

and colder than it need be
for the turtle, and the story
circulates back east again
where Rhoda lives and sets

the law down. *I take the check,*
she says. *You stay upstairs*
except the day the nurse comes in.
Her tale returns to Stan's

and to his metal shed out back
where her boxes molder in the heat.
The saving grace—Stan never takes
a swing at her, no, never once.

Her fear—that Rhoda will.
The story starts the month
her husband died and cycles
to the year in bed and to the valve

that's turned to chalk, to what
those children fight about—
where to put her, how to crack
their mother's calcified old pump.

Jack Coulehan

My Uganda

for Sister Concepta
Najjemba

Sister scans the hills
for burning weeds—
whatever she sees
is Uganda.

She sips lemonade
on the porch steps,
watches the roofs
for menacing birds
and suffers sleeplessness—
sleep is Uganda.

Sister's pale blue habit
is a vista so distant
that barefooted runners
carry tales
across her savannah.

Enveloped by the spoor
of Africa, she sways
and tells tales
of midnight raids
and dead cattle,

her father
shackled to a chair
as they shock him
in the balls,

her brother
necklaced to a tire,
doused with gasoline
and set afire.

When sister speaks
about the tragic fever
that carries her country
out of its senses, her body is
Uganda

While the other sisters
sleep, Uganda sits
at the edge of her bed.

She runs her hands
along her thighs,
she whispers *mai mai*
softer
than the vibrating fan.

Sister's fingers
ripple through the dark.
Her prayer
is medicine, her prayer
is sweet,
sweet medicine.

After Chekhov

Chekhov in a Photograph with Tolstoy, 1901

The old man leans back on the couch,
his right leg curled comfortably
beneath his left thigh. His boots shine
elegantly, but the dark smock
is wrinkled. Two horns of white beard
hang from his querulous face,
suggesting unhappiness. His hat
is sunny, but passion smolders
beneath it—*Get the hell out of here!*

The young man sits straight on the couch,
right leg crossed over left, hands
clasped on his knee, ensuring that he
is properly tucked. Grave in his suit,
he sports a cravat. His hat blocks
the window that opens toward them,
separating the old man's rage
from the other's pique. Chekhov's eyes
above his natty beard don't blink.

Jack Coulehan

Seven Tales

1. Tart

The day before yesterday
I visited the man
whose body this was—

a poet
who lived in a refuge
for the chronically
homeless.

Just before his death
he asked for an apple tart.

I went to the bakery
across the street
and banged on the warm door.

When he saw the tart
he jumped up
and danced on his toes,
wheezing, *The very thing!*

The very thing!
Imagine!

2. Oats

A peasant woman carting rye
fell off her wagon
into a stone culvert
and was horribly injured.

Let the lentils go, Kirila,
she whispered in pain
to her daughter,
do the lentils later,
but now thresh the oats
before frost arrives.

I had morphine
at the tips of my fingers.
Forget the oats, I said,
we need to speak.

But, sir, the oats are ever so good!

3. Chekhov in Greek School

At the beginners' bench in Greek School,
the teacher's cassock swings beside my seat.
I flub the assignment. He twitches
curds of dandruff from his beard. His switch
is less harsh than my father's hand,
but the snickering children are crueler.

Son of a peasant, I'm a failure with Greeks
that lurk at the docks, cracking their knuckles.
Every day the same: mornings at school,
home by noon, work at the shop until late,
keep my mouth shut. Father, who bows
so deeply to the merchant Greeks

he scrapes his forehead, throttles mother
when the soup turns out too salty. On Sunday
he drags me into church for early Mass
with Greeks, who choke on their cuds of holiness.
When my voice rises steeply from the choir,
my father beats his chest in penance.

4. Death Watch

Not that I didn't love him—
but he was a mad dog
of a brother, a thorn in my side.

He'd disappear for months
with his concubine
and emerge on a raft of shit.

What did my brother ever promise
that bore fruit?

Two months at his bedside—
I wandered around his rooms at night
and shuffled my implements.

What was said, was said
a hundred times. What wasn't said
was closer than comfort.

I left at the moment
you would have left him
if you, too, had been there.

When I returned, another brother said,
He died in my arms.
And my sister told me,
I emptied the chamber pot.

When the last rose is gone, my brother lingers.

5. The King of the Medes

Melikhovo, 1893

Dear Lika, you ask me to be serious
and say *I love you*. Well, I'm finished
sucking the breast of Mother Russia.
This autumn the oats are lagging.
Our cook ruined the eggs at breakfast.
The pig snuffles maize in the garden.
Last night the ponies ate the entire
cauliflower patch as we were sleeping.
I purchased a cow for six rubles—
its voice reminds me of my father's.
How scandalous, the King of the Medes
has been reduced to this predicament!
Let's escape to Constantinople
by jumping out the window. I'm not afraid
of the caliph's minions and tattooed
concubines. But I *am* afraid
of saying *Lika, my love, I caress*
your eyelids, I embrace your thighs.
The depth of my desire terrifies me…
Did I tell you about our drunken cook?
Masha is well. Send a note when you can.
Goodbye, my cantaloupe. Anton.

6. Babushka

Melikhovo, 2000

The school that Chekhov built,
a mud-covered village behind it—
decaying huts, knots of birch,
barnyard geese, as skinny
as ferrets. A mosquito marsh.
A babushka, wrapped in an
overcoat with rubber boots,
sits at the door. We pay her
fourteen rubles and scrape mud
from our soles before entering.
In the room Chekhov's sister
taught in—rows of desks
like polished roots and a map
of the yellow world. The woman's
face blames us for being
tourists. A predatory whine
of insects replaces rain.
The vestibule is so damp
babushka's knees honk.
She spends hours alone,
stamping her feet on the floor
to pump their circulation.
She shows us the stack
of spiritual reading
her granddaughter sent
from Moscow. The driver spits,
Babushka!
Her husband drank himself
to death, he says. And she wants
you to know this village
hasn't had a birth in twenty years.

7. Empty Soup

We made a soup last week
from turnips and thistles—
that's how poor we've become.

In the mill, our machinery
is down—we sweep the floor
all week with politics.

Better to be a free man
than a cog—stories like this
are spice for our pot.

In our lives, too—the voice
of the Russian nation
is drab and heroic

like a long family trip
after a death—so much
to do, so little time.

Empty soup—that's what
the woman from Novotny
served for her supper.

Yes, I am grateful,
she said, even for the thistles
in the cracks of my life.

Lovesickness

As real as melancholy, baldness, headache,
and lice. As real as Christ's love for his bride
the Church. As real as an abundance of bile
in the brain's ventricles, tumbling the lover
ever forward with sighs and hidden thoughts.
As real as parched mouth, edematous tongue,
bitterness in the throat, as though the patient
had eaten unripe plums. As real as rapture,
but as pale in complexion as spent humor.

Cures include travel: it diminishes languor
and permits the beloved's image to lessen
in potency. The induction of sleep
by medicinal herbs: this cleans the slate.
Wine, conversation, and reading some books:
these serve as cathartics, purging the patient's
sad obsessions. And litigation
may also be helpful, by putting an edge
on the heart's collapse. In serious cases
these remedies may not be sufficient.
As a last resort, prescribe sexual relations,
following which the illness will relent.

Jack Coulehan

William Carlos Williams Circumcises Hemingway's First Son

So I said, sure, and why not? The next sweet
     morning of Paris
          drunk with the warm scent
of rain on gravel
     in Luxembourg Gardens
          and my head as big as a bucket
a—shall we say— aftereffect
     of the prizefights we went to
          the night before
the four of us
     roiled in the grit and sawdust and sweat
          —*Kill him!*
          Kill the bastard!—Flossie cried.
So I picked up my leather kit and went back
     to Hem's flat
          laid the kid on the kitchen table
and lopped off his foreskin
     —*his teeny binky*, Hadley cried—
          which in those days
was what you did. At the sight of Bumby's blood,
     bloody big Hem
     standing at the side of the table
          holding the kid's head
 collapsed
     a sack of potatoes, a tin of lard
          fainted *ker-boom*
dead to the world. After the days in Paris
     they kept asking me
          how could I go back
to the pale complexities of practice?

To the grime
            of Rutherford's bodies?
The drum of routine—
        I think of Hem on the floor at the first drop
            of blood.
What a man! It isn't anything
        I could explain, I tell them. It's
            making a living.

Jack Coulehan

Astonishment

In memory of John Stone,
poet and physician

John, enthusiasm means possession
by the gods. To chisel the lines, to snap
your clauses into joint, to question
which word is most elegant and apt,
requires patience, detail, craft. But the juice
you pump into their hearts, the baritone
passion of your spleen, your antic voice—
these matter most. Your lungs grown
silent, astonishment still breathes in the lines
of your poems. You said the heart leads, the head
explains. Maybe, but its explanations
leave a lot to be desired. John, the spread
of grace is patchy at best, but your voice
enhances it. *Therefore, let us rejoice.*

He Lectures on Grace

Sewage Treatment

Visiting the sewage treatment plant
beside the Monongahela River
in Pittsburgh—that trip was another
of the million small betrayals
I suffered at the hands of teachers
who didn't comprehend anything
about medicine. I chalked it up
to their obsession with demanding
irrelevance. *Those who can't do, teach.*
Then they put sewage on the exam!

At the time I planned to become
a psychiatrist and later that summer
married my sweetheart, a definite plunge
to maturity. That lush grass,
the continuous thrum of machines.
the clatter of catwalks. A uniformed flunky
took us to each step of purification
from sludged to seraphic. Today,
I'm imagining those pipes and pools
continually refreshed by filtering,
aeration, and slime, enabling
the past to flow into me, more wholesome
and drinkable than when it happened.

Jack Coulehan

Man Mountain Dean

Gorgeous George grimaced across the ring
at Man Mountain Dean, whose belly bulged
like twins beneath his bib. The Mountain
lunged at that pansy's legs, but Gorgeous
swiveled free and flashed his teeth. My grandma
gripped the arms of her chair and grunted
at the Philco screen. *They're faking it,* I nagged
again, but she just glared and worked her dentures.
Gorgeous, in his high-laced boots, goose-
stepped around the ring, spritzing his chest
with perfume, until Man Mountain Dean
torpedoed him. *Damn, you brute!* My grandma
cried—darkness was loosed upon the world.
Protestants marched against the pope
and Adlai Stevenson had gotten in.
Man Mountain Dean, holding aloft
his marvelous belt, threatened the crowd
with his fist. My grandma and the pansy
moaned. She doesn't know the world, I thought
and dropped my book to the davenport
to pass her the dish of mints. I won't be fake,
I told myself, and follow someone's script.

Grease

What he remembers about the pits
under the rolling mills at Wheeling Steel
is that spent grease had no way out
unless lifted through a hatch at the top
by bucket. The hatch was big enough
for a skinny kid to crawl through.
Grease to the calves of his boots, oilskin
glistening with tarry rivulets,
cloying stench, suck of cleaving grease's
surface—With the bucket partly filled,
he tugged a cable for his partner to pull.
The pails were lighter than he expected,
but soon queasiness rose in his caw.
Steel sheets sped thinner and thinner
above his helmet, his spirit buckled
and collapsed beneath its oily sheen,
its brutal power. He struggled to become
smaller, zero, zilch in an atmosphere
as heavy and toxic as Venus.
Eyes cast down, he climbed out of the pit
before his stint was up and hunched
on a bench for the rest of the shift.
Some of the others slapped him on the back
and told him stories. One offered a share
of his thermos. This was the closest
he had ever been to another man.

Jack Coulehan

Why I Am Not a Pathologist

Clumps of vacuoles mire my sight,
no matter how much I jiggle
the slide, or fiddle with focus.
The higher the power, the bigger
the vacuoles, until under oil
they obscure the slide. I switch
to my other eye—the clumps
of malevolence shift. The only
conclusion—bilateral cancer.
My brain sheds layers, loses
its invincible aura. My heart
grows murkier, simmers
with anger and fear. I confess
to my preceptor—melanoma—
and bow before Nemesis.
The professor cocks an eyebrow,
demands I work until the end
of lab, pierces my interior
windows with light, and then
announces, *Congenital*
central sub-capsular cataracts.
Nothing to worry about.
Frozen bubbles I was born with
mirrored and magnified, just
small spots of imperfection, not
a cauldron of death boiling within.

Delicate Procedures

for J. S.

We climb into our booth
at the Hi Lite Diner
and order mixed grill
and barbequed ribs. You
scold me for not showing up
in Vietnam, and I bat
back your paranoia.
You carry your autopsy
instruments. I bring
my stethoscope and scalpel.
You begin with a standard
Y-incision—in a minute
my heart's on the table. I listen
for the scratch of shrapnel
in your posterior lung fields.
You tag my pump for later,
then sever my lungs
and weigh them. I make
an initial cut
under the lip of your left
fifth rib, teasing the shards
of metal embedded there.
We complete our procedures
before the pie arrives. You reckon
you'll wait until we meet again
to get my brain. I hand you
a napkin with bloody shrapnel
from your back and collect
my organs. We split the bill
and shake hands, anxious
to get home and begin
putting ourselves together again.

Jack Coulehan

The Goddess Grabs Me by the Hair

Between lying on my left side
with an anonymous person propping
a bunched blanket against the small
of my back, and the endoscopist

replacing his instrument on a tray,
I expected to recall duration—
sinking, dreams—not that I cared, given
the juice they gave me, and my relief

that my pancreas had survived.
But a gap of thirty two minutes
on the tape! There ought to be
evidence, like a crack in the panel,

or a subtle displacement of carpet.
Not nothing. It isn't, after all,
our older, all-forgiving sister,
sleep, they put us into. It's a

precipice. When the Great Mother surged
to the surface, grasping my head
by its hair, and lopped it over the rim
of consciousness, I was the last to know.

The Little Flower

A nun tugs me by the elbow and scuttles
us back to a tiny room behind her shop—
Praise the Lord, I'm ninety tomorrow—

and fumbles in a box of pamphlets
for the relic, a piece of cardboard
with a swatch of linen stapled on it,

wrapped in plastic. Fabric that once touched
the uncorrupted corpse of St. Theresa,
the Little Flower. All day I've simmered

in the oil of memory. The monastery
reminds me of a past in which holiness
was varnished by cruelty. Crazy,

this midsummer nun is wheedling me
to pray. Whose mistake is it, hers or mine?
I was only looking for a Pepsi

and aspirin, not the story of pain
in her hips, which gets bad when it's damp,
but better when she rubs them with the relic.

Jack Coulehan

In Praise of Virtue

A student twitches in her seat,
irked at my wasting her time.
Fidelity, fortitude, compassion—
what a moldy scent they exude!
She wants content, words cut
from a block of granite, words
built with bricks from the ground up,
not old sheets waving in the wind.
Virtue! No wonder she Googles
an alternate route. Virtue, for her
is either fraudulent, or a track
too deep in the thalamus
to count. Pixel by pixel,
my student fades. *Wait! Wait!*

I'll juggle seven words at once
while walking on stilts.
I'll twist my face into a clown's
to capture her attention,
make her giggle with delight…
Too late. Only a wisp
of her remains. I wanted to warn her
words can grind and abrade.
I wanted to show her the bruises.

Mission of Mercy

A voice in the dark, enroute
to Australia. A pyramid of shadow
in the aisle. Me, climbing, half-asleep,
across a pair of wedged-in bodies
to present my rusty skills, hoping
to help without slipping up. The man,
crumpled between pillows on the floor.
His calm wife, kneeling on an aisle seat,
explains the seizures—rigidity,
posturing, tremor—and raises his arm
to reveal the bracelet. Groggy, but awake.
His pulse, slow and strong. Lips pale, a trace
of vomit. Breathing, quiet. He asks,
What happened? I feel a bolus of relief—
nothing to do now but accept credit
and return to sleep. A round of smiles
and pats, as we ease Mr. McKeever
toward the galley. At which moment
the pulmonologist arrives with his
First Class compartment doctor kit,
whispers his expertise in situations
like this, orders the man down, begins
to insert an intravenous line.
Turn up the lights. Tear off his shirt.
Scurrying. Immediate tension.
Cardiogram. Valium. Saline
solution. Passengers emerge, blinking,
from somnolence. Next thing, I think,
he'll want to resuscitate the guy,
just in case. *Might as well go back to your seat,*
he slaps me *on the* shoulder. *No sense
for both of us to lose a night's sleep.*

Jack Coulehan

He Lectures on Grace

The first setback to his talk
on grace was the lack
of sync between his laptop
and their projector.
An electronic screech
pierced the room, but when
at last they found a man
to fix the sound, it lessened
a little. And the glitch
in his introduction
by a ponderous former dean,
who mistakenly called him
a family doctor from
Missouri, while holding
the podium up with bursts
of hot gas, and then left
for his important meeting
before the talk—that could
have been worse. And the lunch,
a catered spread of salads,
sandwiches, schmoozing,
and lack of attention, didn't
actually prevent him
from speaking. Faces arose,
faces fell, the clatter
resumed. How he relished
this lesson in detachment!
And began, *Courage, said*
Ernest Hemingway
is grace under pressure.

Nesidioblastosis

A fantastic topic! This morning's
Grand Rounds is thoroughly erect
and in the dark! *Nesidio*
appears for the first time without his turban
and uniform, addressing the audience
on enzymes and the Islets in his
dazzling dialect of molecules—
but *Nesidio's* story, his beliefs
about ambiguity and pain, his forging
a pact with forces of destruction,
the body's distress and resistance,
the fine silk pantaloons of *Nesidio's*
culture—all this is lost to listeners,
who struggle with numbness and armor,
and seek evidence of important times
in teeth marks on their Styrofoam cups.
Blastosis. My tongue lingers with reverence
for science and uncertainty about
Nesidio, whose presence this morning
is unaccounted for. A strange little man
with dozens of terminally thin
slices of pancreas. A series
of diagrams that string the tiniest
aphids of life together. Is his
a *nom de guerre?* It's nearly eleven
and none of the scattered, seated bodies
asks a question, even though an awkward
balloon, filled with the bold caption,
BLASTOSIS! has risen above each head
in the room—except two. Some of the balloons
twitch, others divide. No sacred liturgies
this morning, no blessings, and no quips.
Nesidio has done his level best
and now retires. A scent of loneliness
lies in wait. How worn is the felt
on ancient auditorium seats!

Jack Coulehan

Levitation

Bursting with Danger and Music

With my window cracked a little,
a reed of sound penetrates the van,
as the road slashes

through hills of lacquered snow
and unfreezes tiny valves
of fossil crustaceans.

Uncover them! Drape the slopes
with iced instruments—
recorders, mouth harps, oboes, flutes!

In this February snow
I'm bursting with danger and music
I cannot control, O my soul.

Jack Coulehan

To the Man with the Video Camera

at the Monastery on Patmos:
I am the person who followed you
into the gold-encrusted vestment room
where you circled each piece and shot it,
and along the hall of chalices
into the chamber of relics.
On the spiky path to the cave
where St. John went ecstatic,
it was miraculous you didn't trip
on loose rock while filming, or look up
to the breathless Aegean landscape.
You steadied your elbow at the crack
in the rock where God spoke, and filmed
its irregular black mouth
for minutes—the time was much less,
but because of the smirk in my heart,
I exaggerated your crime,
and that of your wife and two children
who stayed near the bus and bought ice cream.
All is forgiven now. To tell you the truth,
when I reach for that monastery,
I need to invent just about
every image, save you and the camera,
which to my way of thinking are solid
historical fact. I wonder if
you've kept that video? Would you send me
a copy?—even a small glimpse
of the vestments, or the empty bus?

Theology

On our trip across the continent
I had intended to explain
what I had learned about God,

but in the back seat the baby
screamed from Saskatoon
to California. When she finally fell

into exhausted silence, I jumped
to the proofs of God's existence,
to which you listened less than a minute.

Whereof we cannot speak,
Wittgenstein wrote,
we must remain silent.

Vermillion streaks above the horizon,
Mount Shasta's darkened symmetry,
the fertile cloak of stillness

I hadn't yet put on. The road
frowned at me like a favorite aunt,
whose grim face twitches

then collapses in laughter.

Jack Coulehan

Midnight Romance

On the midnight train from Moscow to Petersburg
we aim for romance: a milky glass of tea
straight from the samovar, the boreal forest
sliding backward beside our compartment window,
a uniformed steward to serve shots of vodka
for us to knock down, our two pale bodies
tangled on crisp sheets. But we stumble into
an airless sleeper packed with partially dressed
Orthodox priests and their elbows and abdomens,
and an angry conductor twists us into
another car and drops us into berth
6, like stunned turtles in a terrarium.
The French in #5 and the pair of Texans
whose #7 is dirtier than their horses' stalls
rub broken glass into their grief outside our door.
We just aim for relief, but giant mosquitoes
prick us, especially you, and the toilet's odor
is heavier than virtue, and our attendant
smokes behind a newspaper in his seat. Shall I ask
about the comfortable climate control
in the brochure? Or mention the lack of towels
to the tank-like woman who barks at him?
And you promise me—with twelve volcanic bites
and your face already swollen—
you'll die of anaphylaxis before we arrive.
Why doesn't anything work? You insist that I
or the repellant, equally impotent,
smash something, anything. The embedded sweat
of thousands of Soviets seeps from every surface
and surges against our window. Wrapped in
woolen blankets right up to our faces, we eat
the last of the cheese and granola bars. The train
shudders and a voice announces in Russian,
Attention! Romance is about to begin.

A Theory of Labor

for Elizabeth Rose

For the seventeenth hour
you heave and sweat,
stretched, but stuck.
Your pelvic floor
is faltering, its muscles
ripping. Collin
butts his head against
desire, a drum you share.
It's old news our openings
are disproportionate
to needs. What sense
does labor make?
Look at the swift
appearance of apes
into this Garden
of Paradise. Daughter.
you'd think by now
God would have given up
his pique about our taste
of that forbidden fruit
and softened your bed
with roses.

Jack Coulehan

Toenails

Plasters of fungus, horny planks
of keratin, replace the toenails
that never meant a whit to me
until they thickened and went gray.

The podiatrist shrugs with indifference
at their display. *Consider the length*
and burdens of treatment, he muses.
It's true my toenails spend their days

encased in shoes, so why attempt
to salvage their integrity? My body
blossoms with dozens of losses,
each more convincing than the last,

so why waste enthusiasm
on pink, pliable nails, when I could
spend it on a younger, steadier heart,
a deeper, more distinguished face?

Pedal hope—a quest proportionate
to my place in the world, the way
of the Tao, awaiting some small life
to poke its chin from the stony ground.

The Five Moons of Venus

My married sons, who went out on a whim
with a telescope that neither of them
had figured out, set it up in a spot
near the barn, where the leaves were thin.

There was lunacy about their game,
but not mine. I was in a daze
from chasing grandkids when they came in—
We've sighted the five moons of Venus!

I pulled on boots. A crescent hung
among the stars. With the scope I could
demonstrate Orion, my only trick,
and they showed me an orange unblinking orb

shining in a gap between the trees
and around it a spoke of four white specks—
Jupiter! And its four moons that didn't fit
the scheme and set Galileo thinking

that God might be more complicated than
we imagine and less like a larger
version of us. How much of the known
might be wrong! How much of the truth hidden!

Jack Coulehan

Sweetness

I notice a woman's shoe,
fluorescent pink, wedged
to its back between rocks.

The Saturday afternoon
of clean-up. Cub Scouts
scour the beach for trash.

Parts of plastic forks,
Styrofoam cups,
a long, ragged wound

of kelp and worn grass.
Restoration—when
the woodcock and martin

arrive to begin breeding,
this time they'll find
a sweet beach. Scouts,

trailing plastic bags, earn
their badge. Fingers, branches,
stones, a knife—I pry,

twist, dig, sculpt the shoe
from its tomb, until
suddenly the suck gives. Free!

A pink shoe! Put this moment
toward sweetness, add it
to the pages of hope.

Phrenology

Concavities and bumps above my ear
speak narratives I never would have known
before relentless loss of all my hair

turned truth about my scalp so baldly clear—
the story of my life is in the bone.
Convexities and slumps above my ear

identify the site of passion: here.
Like tenacity and hope, it's in a zone
invisible before the loss of hair

writ large the heady script of character.
Depression, fancy, awkwardness intone
complexity that's bunched above my ear

for you to read. Your gentle fingers, dear,
interpret my desire and mine alone.
My scalp is blessed to have no trace of hair.

It shines with gratitude—I love your care
for this old scalp, though never have I won
a way to read the bumps above *your* ear,
which even now are swathed in silver hair.

Jack Coulehan

Snoring

possesses me in the dark of bed.
My brain buzzes as much as ever,
but undercover, an electric tread
has slipped its gears. In sleeping I sever
my narrative, anticipate silence—
but what do you know? A provocative din
replaces me in bed, its violence
drives you mad. At Pandemonium
in Milton's hell—I drag alarming groans
across the rocks. I snuffle in the trough.
I imitate a whale. No wonder you soon
sleep in another room. I used to scoff
at men, whose troubled sleep came close
to suffocation, as if it were their choice.

Cosmic Sonnets

1.

A spasm of loneliness grips my
esophagus—I wish it were otherwise.
On my side of the phone, the lousy
old forest sinks into darkness and silence.
On your side, the illuminated kitchen
blazes with liveliness, and in the hum
of your eager voice, I imagine
a slim piece of our separation
sawed off and the two ends brought nearer
together. I see us as Siamese twins,
joined at the chest, sharing one heart. I fear we're
predictable, dated, and too damn
intense, which leads me to contemplate
just how our beginnings made us that.

2.

What does a Big Bang mean? A speck
an astronomer picked up has spent thirteen
billion years in transit. They accept
it as a type of relic from the time
the universe spun from a thin ocean
of monotony to the lumpiness
that created *things*. The scent of lotion
on your hands, the unintended caress
of your fingertips brushing my lower arm,
my gratitude at spinning in an orbit
that nurtures life, your well worn alarm
when I ask questions like, Does any of it
mean anything? Or are we going anywhere?
I don't know, but please stay, until we're there.

3.

The bang couldn't have been *big*. Dimension
didn't exist until the event
had occurred; nor, for that matter, time.
In retrospect, after a moment
had elapsed, the bang had to be minimal,
a *ping*, since ten to the minus ten of space
was all there was. We struggle with scale
in love as well. We think: How ardent the chase!
How deep! How eternal! But I've noticed
our conversations are sparser than they were
and quieter. As you sit in the Lotus
position, across from my computer
desk, you're bathed in glorious photons, *ping*,
oblivious to the original Bang.

4.

In the first ten to the minus eleven
of the universe's story, the plot
was complete, its dramatic tension
a sham. But the fact is, we have yet
to decipher the text. In the Theory
of Everything, we've lost at least seven
dimensions along the way—fairy
universes. Only the brushfire of time
and the trinity that makes up space
remain: quasars, stars, and planets where
we live, but your presence, my love, creates
a twelfth—yet first—dimension, a rare
unbroken symmetry—call it *Dance*—
which enlivens space and time and chance.

Levitation

If I'm lucky—which is to say, not tied
to rehearsing the day's mistakes,
or imagining myself vindicated,
or receiving a prize for devoting
my life to service—I levitate.
My dinosaur brain turns into a bird.
I wave to the guards at Aspinwall School
and skip like a girl on the path
between First and Emerson. How normal
it feels to gravitate upwards, to skim
across tops of the weeds, to shed my
dejection and awkwardness, and to ride
the maelstrom almost, but not quite, safely.

Natural History

Grackles

How many grackles live in the ceiling
above my room? As a rule, the deadbeats
are not communal, but the skittering
that threatens my refuge is surely
the making of more than one ruffian bird
and her brood. Those muscle-bound grackles
bully the five or six acres of woods
in back of the house still allowed to exist
as long as the county authority
owns them. Those dive-bombing terrorists,
they're out of the garbage and into their own
waste, their own niche in my consciousness,
those birds are insouciant and alien
to the big picture and good intentions
and the virtue of discipline. Those grackles
have spattered the space above my room,
reminding me how vulnerable I am.

Jack Coulehan

Do No Harm

Lights on. A spider in the sink is stunned.
Big sucker, hairy, brown. The body
bulges. Otherwise, it's squat. If I stand
a minute without moving, it'll glide
across the porcelain, attending
to its needs. Why do spiders appear?
This one lowered itself on a thread
that's gone. Exploring? It couldn't have been.
Spiders don't. Attracted to moisture?
The sink's dry now, but vulnerable
to flood. This arachnid is as good as dead.
What kind of being? I have no way
of understanding how it feels. It may eat
its own eggs. It hasn't friends. The sheen
of the porcelain means nothing to it.
Act without thought. I will turn the tap
to the left and pull out my razor.
Shouldn't I snap off the light and wait
for the spider to leave? Or flick it
gently with a Kleenex? I don't. I let
the torrent loose and turn to the shower,
so I can't see the spider struggling
and sliding on porcelain. For all I know
its whole life flashes in front of it.

Predators

On a Sunday morning behind the house
on Resaca Street, a falcon pecks
what's left of a pigeon, a disk
of white feathers on the grass, a scene
I hadn't counted on for breakfast.

As the year runs out, there's only a pane
of window between my newspaper's
Afghanistan! and the tense
black predator. She's edgy as I am.
Can she sense my alien stare,

my questioning? Immiscibility mixed—
terror and peace, hers and mine, falcon
and pigeon, clear and ambiguous,
looked at and looking; immersion,
irony; predator, prey; pleasure

and pain. She worries her glob of flesh
again—but tightens, jerks and drops it.
A threatening quiet. She senses
a world going wrong, a predator—
or just my eyes' pressure? The falcon

impales the remains of her pigeon.
Without holding back, or bandying about,
or calling forth the baggage of virtue,
she bolts to a perch at the top of the fence
and vanishes.

Jack Coulehan

Darwin's Barnacles

After five years mulling about finches
and tortoises, he knew that perfection
was a product of chance. What next, he asked?
It wasn't long before the migraines came
and forced him to slow down. Whom could he trust
with the manuscript? How much suffering
would his theory cause? He dissected
the smallest barnacles in the world,
mere specks of creatures. Strangely, in one
the male was a miniscule parasite
that spent its whole life in the flesh
of the female. Could this be a mistake?
What kind of a God would have chosen to create
a species like that, in which the male
was nothing but a degenerate,
larva-like sac with a sex organ?
Darwin asked himself, had the time come,
finally, to explain the simple truth?
The ill-formed little monster—to which he gave
the name *Ibla cumingii*—
was every bit as perfect as man.

Natural History

About survival the trees of Australia
have it right. Hang in. Don't waste moisture
on beauty. Don't worry about the next
romantic bloke who wants to be inspired
by the landscape. Don't spread your foliage
for pleasure, but hunker into the cracks
for the long haul. Thicken your leaves
to lessen the surface. Polish them
tight and hard like fried chips. If you need to,
strangle the life from a few of your limbs
until they whiten and drop. The maroon stain
of sap you splay across the tortured trunk
of your body is not a calamity.
Regarding survival, ugliness
is a blessing. That which stands alone, fits in.

Jack Coulehan

The Invention of Language

Eve hadn't intended to become
the mother of anyone, let alone
all of us, by making crazy sounds.

The woman who invented language
repeated her words time after time,
which unsettled her clan.

She persisted in playfulness
long after her body grew round
and her whimsy should have gone.

Not that the woman who invented
language didn't dig for grubs
like everyone else and lengthen

her man's disposition
by rubbing against him,
but in addition

she catapulted from *skins-warm-
skin* to *clothing* and invented *time*
by keeping track of her blood

by the cycling moon.
What poured from her mouth
was troubling. The clan had no needs

not met by whistle and croak.
No wonder they balked at the woman
whose frenzy was metaphor.

Mungo Woman

New South Wales

Bones embedded in the dunes
of an ancient lake, in a land
once full of sisters and cousins:
insects, their calcified pupae
stuck in transit from life
to fluttering death;
oysters, their opalescent shells
long dimmed; skeletons
of fish, whose knuckles of ear bones
listen to forty thousand years
of dry wind.

So this is the afterlife: bones
baked bronze and burnt umber
in a gutted bed. She knelt
in reeds next to the shore,
her hands cupped with water,
unaware
her next sip would be endless.

Jack Coulehan

Yellow Jacket

for Lisa Cairns

What about the wasps
that invade our space
and harvest our lunch
for their nest? One
works on remnants
of cheese. A second zips
melon to baguette
and back. A third alights
on a gob of ham, half
pearly fat, the size
of a bean. Why does she
so dampen our delight?

She works her mandibles
in fat, severs a piece
as big as her thorax
and abdomen. Stricken
by the weight of her load,
she struggles for flight,
her victory glorious.
but damaging—she,
who never left a loose
end, never performed
an ambiguous act. Wasp,
I award you the purple heart.
Now get out.

Cockroach

She carried roaches across the continent
in her backseat, securely stacked in cartons
scrawled *Don't Tip,* trays lined with newspaper
moist enough to last for several weeks,
an eternity to a roach. This is much
more than I want to learn,
but she suffers from cancer, and I listen.

On a vacation in Barbados,
she noticed the bugs were not only
more speckled and slower than the ones
she grew up with, but big enough to use
in experiments. Forty years later
she knows more about roaches than anyone
in the world, but now she's leaving it.

In roach language, communication
never breaks down. The pheromones
that link them never lie. In what voice
will I speak when she asks? Her passion
for clarity puts my mistaken signals
to shame. She's built her life around
the carapace of roaches' virtue—
crisp integrity. *They'll long outlast us,*
she remarks. *I have no fears. And no regrets.*

Jack Coulehan

Quetzal

After the archeologist's
daughter ran from the unit,
sobbing, he blinked his eyes
and half-whispered—a finger
plugging the moist tube
that pierced his neck—had I heard
of the quetzal? He spit-balled
the word *Resplendent!*
to the railing. Once,
at his dig near Copan,
a quetzal alighted
on a mound of debris,
dead still, and gazed at him,
a blessing, before it sprang
into the oppressive
green canopy. A golden
feather drifted to his feet.
The Maya were astonished
at the gift. *And ever since,*
he whispered. *Ever since…*
The archeologist's voice
slid from its perch and slipped
into the jungle of tubes
that quickly engulfed him.

Vacancy

At dawn the neon YES
blinks its red eye
at the almost empty lot
in Rushville, Nebraska.

Tumbling from the west,
a *luuuuuing* of cattle
rolls the deserted streets
of asphalt and dust.

A slow train is advancing
its sound. The drone
of a single-engine plane.
A stampede of dogs

at the heels of YES,
YES that bursts through
Nebraskaland Motel's
27 numbered doors

YES the prairie rolls
YES the warm breeze
YES a hoarse wave of cattle
YES its *luuuuuu* unsleeping YES!

About the Author

Physician, poet, and medical educator, Jack Coulehan is currently a Senior Fellow of the Center for Medical Humanities, Compassionate Care, and Bioethics at Stony Brook University. He has written extensively about communication, empathy, and literature in medicine, and the role of poetry in healing. Jack co-edited two anthologies of poems by physicians, *Blood & Bone* and *Primary Care*; and previous collections of his own poetry include *First Photographs of Heaven*, *The Heavenly Ladder*, and *Medicine Stone*.

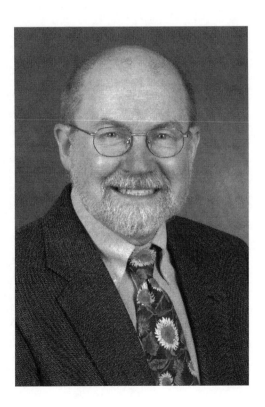